MANAGEMENT OF BREAST CANCER AND (PRBC)

BREAST CANCER DURING PREGNANCY

Medical Education Series

By: S Sabri

Table of Contents

Preface 1

1) Algorithm for Breast lump during Pregnancy 4
2) Breast Anatomy 5
3) Breast Triple Assessment 6
4) Breast Quadrants 6
5) Breast Clinical Proforma 7
6) Breast Imaging.. 7

Breast lesion biopsy 9

Sterotactic Core biopsy 10

Surgery 11

1) Mastectomy 12
2) Surgery to lymph nodes 13
3) Position of pregnant breast cancer patient during surgery 14
4) Fetal wellbeing monitoring.. 14
5) Is it safe to continue pregnancy during breast cancer? 15
6) Improve Outcome with termination of pregnancy............. 15
7) Can I receive chemo during pregnancy? 16
8) Can I feed breasts during Chemotherapy?....................... 17
9) Can I receive Radiotherapy during pregnancy?............... 17
10) Risk factors for Radiotherapy 18
11) Hormonal Treatment during breast cancer 19
12) Could antiemetics or steroids be used during pregnancy? 21
13) Breast Reconstruction.. 21
14) Can breast cancer affect babies?..................................... 22

References 23

Preface

I was inclined to write about breast cancer as well as the rare condition of breast cancer during pregnancy once our team had an encounter with one of these cases. Along with the management of cases, a lot of literature search was involved in providing the right guidance.

It is a rare condition, and Randomized controlled trials are not possible. Hopefully, going through the document there will be more clarifications and decision making is easy for the patients.

Are the issues very vital, Carry on pregnancy? Can chemo be used? Am I suitable for Radiotherapy? Can I breast feed? What about my future pregnancy? Best time of breast reconstruction? Use of Antiestrogen? How long should I consider contraception?

I have tried to template it in a way that the most common clinical scenarios, questions can be answered in the best possible way.

Special Thanks
Muhammad Aamir
Areej / Areeb

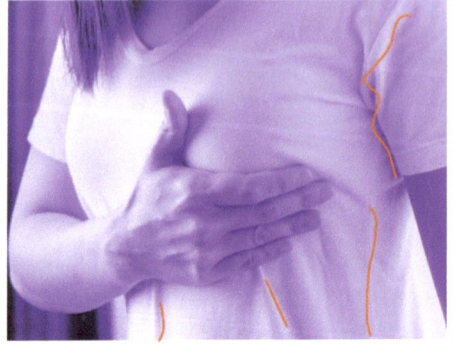

Presentation of new breast lump

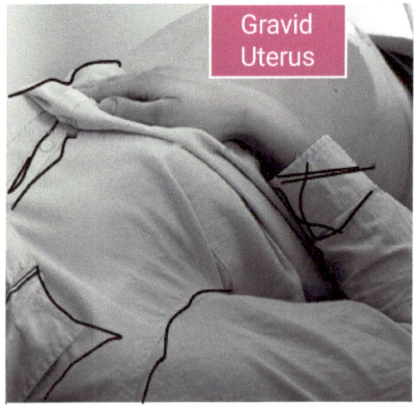

New breast lump in advance pregnancy

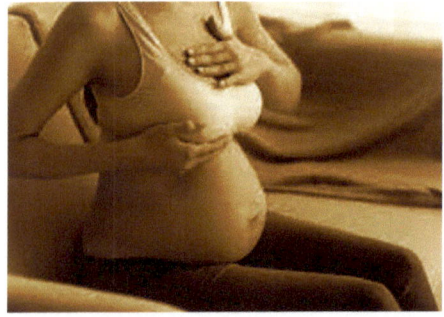

New Breast lump and gravid uterus

Pregnancy related breast cancer

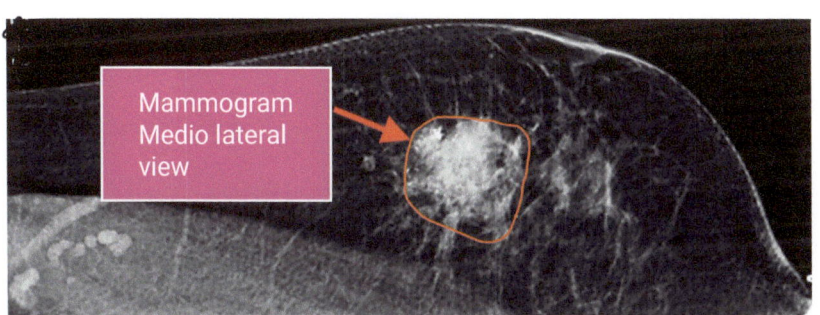

Mammogram Medio lateral view

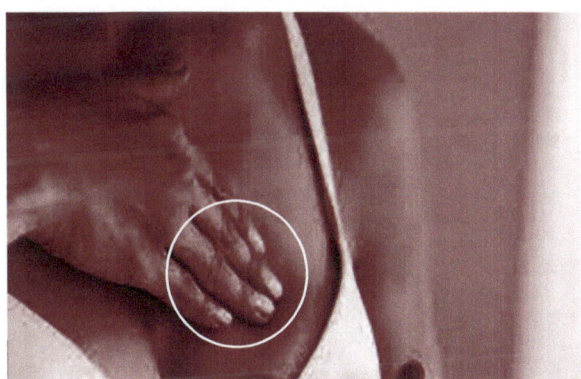

Breast lump upper inner quadrant on left side

1) Algorithm for Breast lump during Pregnancy

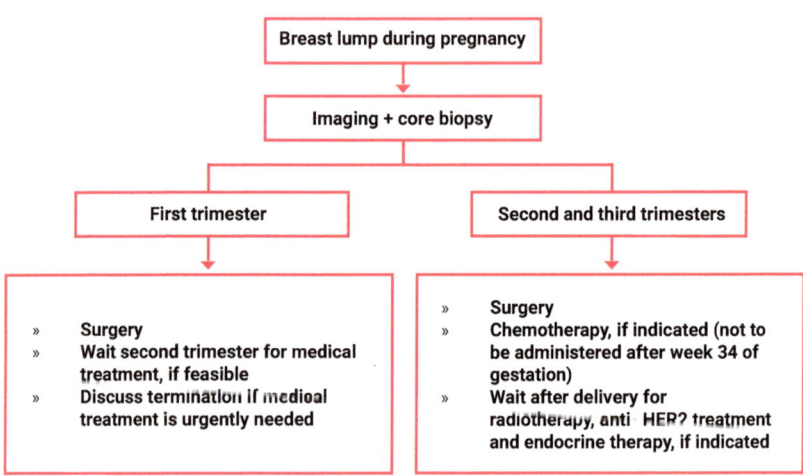

Pregnancy related breast cancer

2) Breast Anatomy

The breasts lie on top of the chest wall and over the pectoral muscles. They contain glands, lobules, fatty tissue, and other structures. Primary breast cancer is breast cancer that has not gone beyond the breast or lymph node (glands) under the arm(axilla).

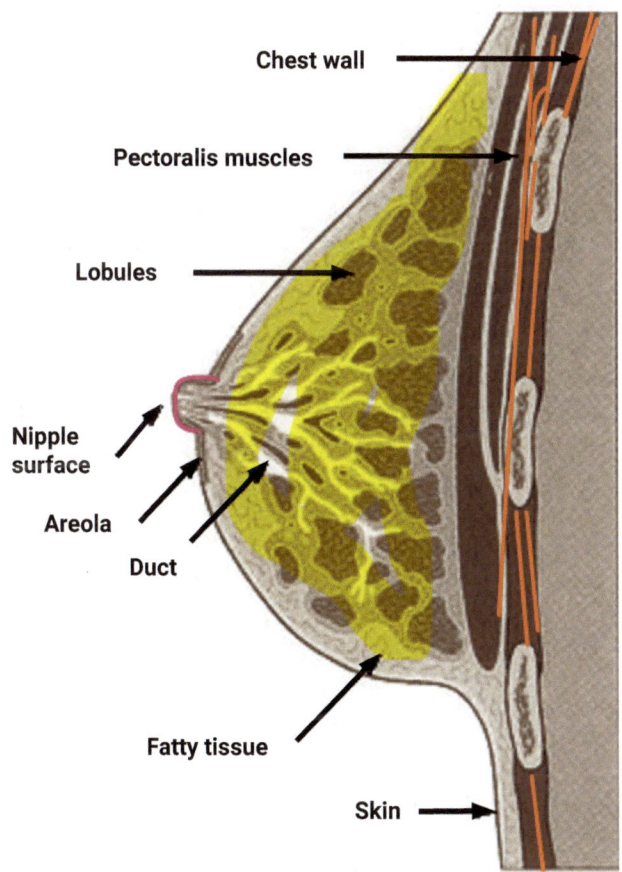

3) Breast Triple Assessment

A triple assessment for breast cancer involves

- Physical examination,
- Scanning of the breasts and
- If necessary, a biopsy

People with suspected breast cancer referred to specialist services are offered the **triple diagnostic assessment** in a single hospital visit.

4) Breast Quadrants

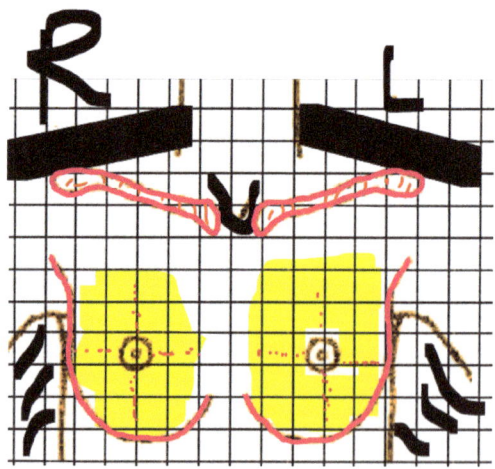

The breast can be separated into 4 quadrants: the upper-outer quadrant (UOQ), upper inner quadrant (UIQ), lower-outer quadrant (LOQ) and lower-inner quadrant (LIQ. The most common site for the occurrence of breast cancer is the upper outer quadrant; the upper inner quadrant is the second site, and both the lower outer and the lower inner quadrants are in the third place.

5) Breast Clinical Proforma

In breast clinics, breast physicians or surgeons will assess you as follows before any investigations will be requested.

- **P1** refers to normal findings.
- **P2** refers to Probably benign (non-cancerous).
- **P3** refers to indeterminate but most likely benign findings. These are discussed in Multidisciplinary team where oncologist, breast surgeon, and radiologist, breast care nurses sit together.
- **P4** refers to findings suspicious of cancer.
- **P5** refers to the presence of **cancer.**

6) Breast Imaging

Ultrasound

Breast ultrasound is the first imaging modality of primary tumour assessment and staging of regional and supraclavicular lymph nodes this is complemented by Mammography supplemented by MRI in selective cases.

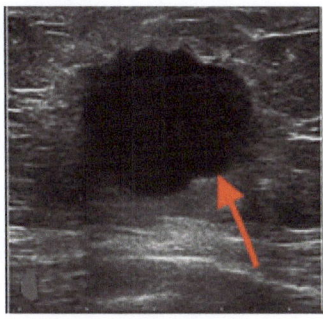

Suspicious breast lesion on ultrasound and biopsy is indicated

Mammogram

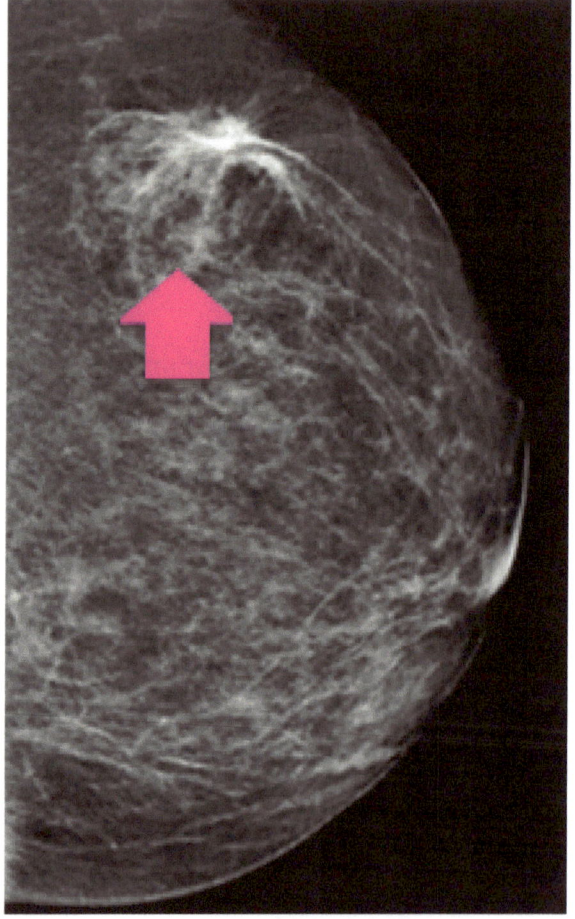

Suspicious lesion on breast mammogram cranio-cadual view

Pregnancy related breast cancer

Breast lesion biopsy

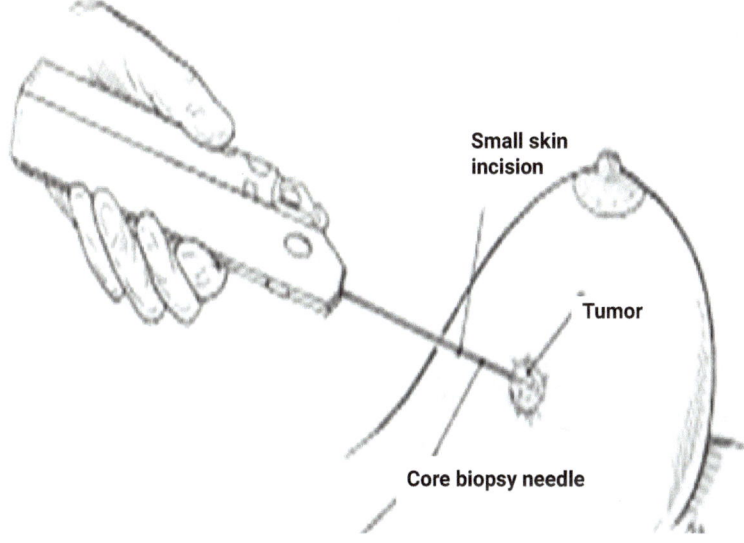

- A core biopsy (also called core needle biopsy) uses a hollow needle to get a sample of breast tissue. **The core biopsy technique is same in pregnant and non pregnant patients.**

Sterotactic Core biopsy

This helps locate the exact position of the area to biopsy. Images of the breast are taken from two different angles to help guide the needle to the precise location. The technique is same in pregnant and non pregnant patients.

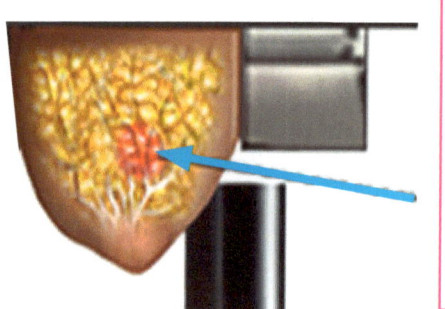

Patient lying flat on couch with breast hanging down

A sample of tissue is taken using a needle biopsy device connected to a mammogram machine and linked to a computer

TREATMENT FOR PRIMARY BREAST CANCER IN PREGNANCY

Surgery

Breast-Conserving Surgery

The aim of breast conserving surgery is to keep as much of the breast while ensuring the cancer has been completely removed; this is also called as lumpectomy or wide local excision. The surgical principle is same for pregnant or non-pregnant patients except anesthetic precautions.

The breast conserving surgery is combined with sentinel lymph node biopsy. If sentinel lymph node does not contain cancer cells no more lymph node is harvested.

In non-pregnant patients the surgical principles are same.

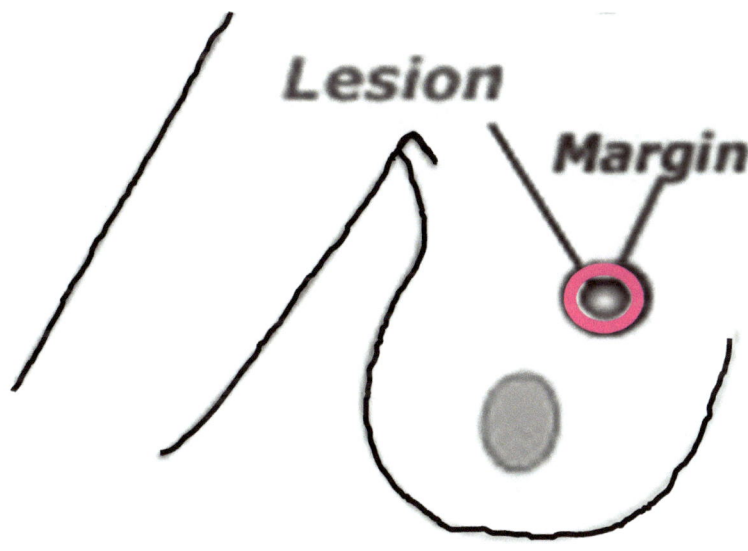

Right breast lesion excised with disease free margin

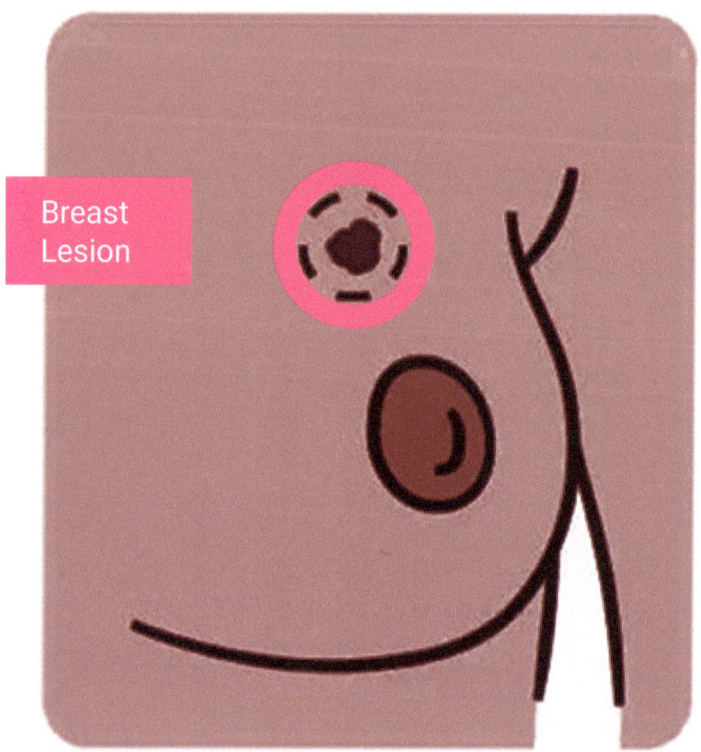

1) Mastectomy

A simple mastectomy is removal of all the breast tissue including skin and nipple area, Mastectomy is usually combined with breast reconstruction. The details to be discussed with pregnant patients and risk, benefits to be individually calculated.

Mastectomy is further divided into **skin sparing type or nipple sparing type.**

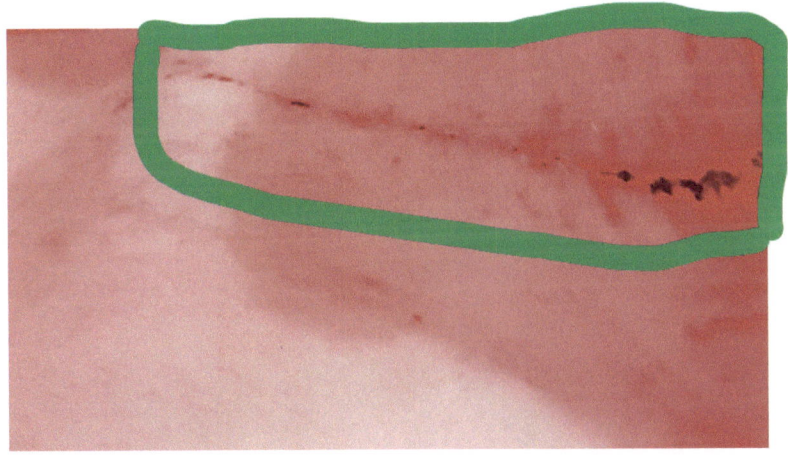

Mastectomy scar showing flat chest wall

2) Surgery to lymph nodes

The lymph nodes are at 3 different levels, the exact location and number of lymph nodes will vary from person to person. lymph nodes. Surgical principles are the same for pregnant and non-pregnant patients.

Lymphedema risk is same in pregnant as well as non-pregnant patients.

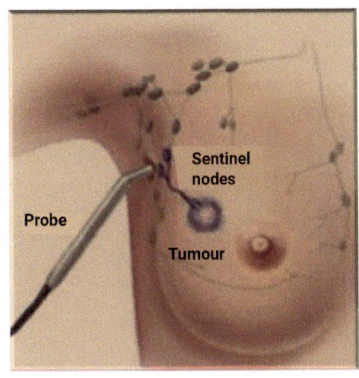

Blue dye or Matrace can not be use in pregnant patient for wide local excision or axillary clearance , Sentinel lymph node is the first lymph node in which breast cancer spreads, low dose technetium can be used for lymph node biopsy.

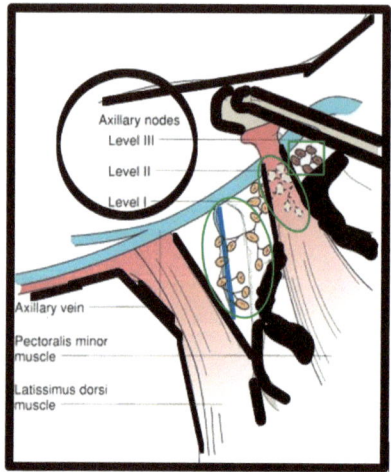

Axillary clearance

Level 1..........Lateral to pectoralis minor.

Level 2........Behind to pectoralis minor.

Level 3.......Medial to pectoralis minnor.

3) Position of pregnant breast cancer patient during surgery

Pregnant patient after 20 weeks of gestation should be positioned with left uterine displacement and adequate maternal oxygenation and optimal utero placental perfusion.

4) Fetal wellbeing monitoring

Fetal wellbeing is assessed before and after breast cancer surgery by close involvement of obstetric team and radiology department to perform the relevant scan before and after surgery.

5) Is it safe to continue pregnancy during breast cancer?

Termination of a pregnancy is not usually recommended by surgeons when breast cancer is diagnosed. Majority of women continue their pregnancy while having breast cancer treatment. However, some women choose not to continue the pregnancy. The decision to terminate a pregnancy is a very personal one. It involves family discussion, obstetric and surgical team and breast care nurse involvement.

6) Improve Outcome with termination of pregnancy

There's no evidence to suggest a termination will improve the outcome for women with breast cancer during pregnancy. However, a termination may be discussed if chemotherapy is recommended during the first 12 weeks (first trimester) of pregnancy. This is the case in secondary breast cancer. Secondary breast cancer is when cancer cells spread from the breast to other parts of the body.

7) Can I receive chemo during pregnancy?

Patients have a lot of questions related to their cancer and pregnancy. One of the important questions is guidance related to any chemotherapy. Chemotherapy destroys cancer cells using anticancer drugs.

First Trimester	Systemic chemotherapy is contraindicated in first trimester because of high rate of fetal abnormalities.
Second Trimester	Chemotherapy is safe from the second trimester and it should be offered according to protocols.
Third Trimester	Chemotherapy can also be used in third trimester as well.

In non-pregnant patients a different approach and chemotherapeutic agents are followed. Chemotherapy can be given before surgery called primary or neoadjuvant chemotherapy or chemotherapy can be given after surgery and before radiotherapy known as adjuvant treatment.

Pregnancy related breast cancer

8) Can I feed breasts during Chemotherapy?

If you were breast feeding when you were diagnosed with breast cancer, your breast surgeon team will recommend you stop breast feeding.

You'll be advised not to breast feed during and for some time after chemotherapy. This is because the chemotherapy drugs can pass to your baby through breast milk. If a patient is towards the end of their chemotherapy they may want to express milk. But expressing milk means patients still be able to produce milk to breast feed after they finish chemotherapy.

9) Can I receive Radiotherapy during pregnancy?

Radiotherapy uses carefully measured and controlled high energy x-rays to destroy any cancer cells that might be left behind in the breast and surrounding area after surgery.

Pregnancy and Trimesters	Radiotherapy is contraindicated in all 3 trimesters until it is lifesaving or preserve the organ function.

Radiotherapy in non-pregnant patients starts a few weeks after surgery and recommended not only for the nodes in armpit area but also the lymph node on either side of breast bone called as internal mammary chain.

10) Risk factors for Radiotherapy

Radiotherapy is not free of risks and predisposes to following:

- Miscarriage
- Teratogenicity
- Microcephaly (Small head)
- Foetal growth restriction
- Mental retardation
- Learning difficulties
- Induction of childhood malignancies
- Haematological disorders (blood disorders)
- Foetal death

11) Hormonal Treatment during breast cancer

The hormonal agents include

- **Tamoxifen**
  In pregnant women, tamoxifen and its metabolites interact with embryonic and fetal tissues, which may lead to teratogenicity. If any hormonal treatment is required, it usually begins after childbirth if ER +ve.

- **Anastrozole**
  Anastrozole is a hormone therapy drug used to treat breast cancer in women who have gone through a natural menopause.

- **Letrozole**
  Letrozole is a hormone therapy drug used to treat breast cancer in women who've gone through a natural menopause (when periods stop).

- **Exemestane**
  Exemestane is a hormone therapy drug used to treat breast cancer in women who have gone through a natural menopause. (when periods stop).

Biological Therapies

Targeted therapy blocks the growth and spread of cancer, Example of targeted therapies for HER 2 positive breast cancer includes Trastuzumab, Pertuzumab, Neratinib. Biological therapies can start after childbirth.

Trastuzumab

Trastuzumab is not recommended during pregnancy as it can affect amniotic fluid levels, and this can potentially affect the baby.

Pertuzumab

Trastuzumab-Pertuzumab can increase the risk of preterm birth, which may lead to various health problems for the newborn.

Neratinib

Taking neratinib while pregnant may be harmful to a developing baby. Some women can still get pregnant even if their periods are irregular or have stopped.

Bisphosphonates

They are given to people who are at risk of osteoporosis. decreased fetal bone growth and accumulation of the drugs in fetal bone. 3-5 They hypothesized that decreased bone growth might be responsible for the decreased fetal weight.

12) Could antiemetics or steroids be used during pregnancy?

Ondansetron, metoclopramide and steroids are commonly used for prevention and treatment. Methylprednisolone or prednisolone are the steroids of choice.

13) Breast Reconstruction

- There are different treatment options available for breast reconstruction, your breast surgeon and breast care nurse will explain which one is likely to suit your best.
- Breast reconstruction at the time of surgery (immediate reconstruction) is not usually offered during pregnancy. Reasons include a higher risk of bleeding during pregnancy and minimizing the time under general anesthetic.
- Breast reconstruction will generally be offered later (delayed reconstruction).
- Delayed breast reconstruction surgery may begin weeks, months or even years after you have completely healed from mastectomy.

14) Can breast cancer affect babies?

There's no evidence that having breast cancer during pregnancy affects your baby's development in the womb. You cannot pass cancer on to your baby. And there's no evidence that your child will develop cancer in later life because you had breast cancer while pregnant.

References

1. Boeri I, Look C, Portman's P, Kipper L, Painter R, Veda Heuvel-Eibrink MM, Am ant F. Breast cancer during pregnancy: epidemiology, phenotypes, presentation during pregnancy and therapeutic modalities. Best Pact Res Clan Oster Gynaecol. 2022 Jun; 82:46-59. Doe: 10.1016/j.bpobgyn.2022.05.001. Pub 2022 May 9. PMID: 35644793.

2. Amouzegar Hashem F. Radiotherapy in Pregnancy-Associated Breast Cancer. Adv. Expo Med Biol. 2020; 1252:125-127. Doe: 10.1007/978-3-030-41596-9_16. PMID: 32816271.

3. Proussaloglou EM, Blanco LZ Jr, Siziopikou KP. Updates in the pathology of Pregnancy Associated Breast Cancer (PABC). Pathol Res Pract. 2023 Apr; 244:154413. Doe: 10.1016/j.prp.2023.154413. Pub 2023 Mar 11. PMID: 36921545.

4. Harvey SC, Mullen LA. The Importance of Understanding Breast Cancer in Pregnancy. J Women's Health (Larch). 2019 Jun; 28(6):737-738. Doe: 10.1089/jwh.2018.7622. Pub 2019 Mar 13. PMID: 30864891.

5. Maxwell CV, Al-Shelli H, Parrish J, D'Souza R. Breast Cancer in Pregnancy: A Retrospective Cohort Study. Gynecology Oster Invest. 2019; 84(1):79-85. Doe: 10.1159/000493128. Pub 2018 Sep 14. PMID: 30219806.

6. Johansson ALV, Stensheim H. Epidemiology of Pregnancy-Associated Breast Cancer. Adv. Expo Med Biol. 2020; 1252:75-79. Doe: 10.1007/978-3-030-41596-9_9. PMID: 32816264.

7. Langer AK. Breast Imaging in Pregnancy and Lactation. Adv. Expo Med Biol. 2020; 1252:17-25. Doe: 10.1007/978-3-030-41596-9_3. PMID: 32816258.

8. Pyle C, Hill M, Sharif S, Fortson C, Shay R. Pregnancy-associated Breast Cancer: Why Breast Imaging During Pregnancy and Lactation Matters. J Breast Imaging. 2023 Nov 30; 5(6):732-743. Doe: 10.1093/jib/wbad074. PMID: 38141239.

www.ingramcontent.com/pod-product-compliance
Lightning Source LLC
Chambersburg PA
CBHW040306220526

45473CB00002B/591